Self Development

And

Inspiration For Success

Written By

Max Samn

Copyright © 2018

ISBN: 9781723811869

Content

Chapter 1

Meaning of a Happy and Successful life

We as a whole have framed our own particular meanings of bliss ideal from adolescence. A considerable measure of these observations are a direct result of adapted improvement i.e. they are a piece of our propensities because of dreary teaching by guardians, instructors, and the general public when all is said in done. That is the reason, none of us has really considered about what precisely fulfills us feel! This inclination has been left to our sub-still, small voice and we basically feel the bliss as per the circumstance we are in.

A ton of little things can offer joy to us. For example, simply the prospect of shopping or burning through cash has a tendency to energize us and fulfills us feel. Openings and new thoughts likewise similarly affect us. This energized state influences us to envision things identified with these episodes. For instance: the viewpoint of taking some time off while getting an office reward would make us energized, as well as make our arrangement and envision the occasion. Indeed, we would feel the ecstasy without really being on the get-away itself! Nonetheless, while being on the genuine get-away, the fervor tends to settle down as one feels mollified.

Same is the situation with objects. We are very insane to buy the most recent mobile phone, workstation, I-case or the new auto. Be that as it may, once we claim that stuff, the fervor settles down and the interest doesn't remain the same. The cycle of energy starts again when another new item is propelled.

How about we stop for a second here and truly consider our space of bliss. Is it related to obtaining the most recent protests as it were? Does it end at wishes being satisfied? Is our space of satisfaction constrained to investing great energy with family or companions as it were? We are so engaged with this cycle of wishes that we really neglect to perceive what genuine joy is and how it very well may be accomplished.

The space or meaning of joy shifts for each person as they have their own particular individual needs. For a few people, accomplishing a decent vocation way gives satisfaction. For a few, it is their satisfaction of objectives and goals whereas expediting bliss the substance of the denied can give a few people joy.

In any case, everyone doesn't have it simple in this world. Our salary, instruction, family, condition, society, and companions all influence our space of satisfaction. We may not generally have the coveted wage expected to satisfy the desires or might be the vocation isn't going as smooth as we had arranged. So what does it do to us? Does it burst our inflatable of expectation and fervor or does it restore our expectations, makes us unmistakable our dreams and set ahead for the future with new inspiration? How would you respond when things don't turn out as you had arranged? Above all, is your response proper or do you have to change your demeanor and observation?

This book is about 'you' and how you can change measurements keeping in mind the end goal to look forward to a superior future. The up and coming parts are an entire guide with the goal that you can set yourself toward another path. All things considered, achievement is tied in with having the correct change in perspective!.

Chapter 2

Objective setting

Objective setting is a vital angle for anybody to be effective. Objective setting empowers you to accomplish your assignments in a sorted out manner and inside the restricted time period. Hence, it is vital that objectives are set precisely. Appropriate arranging is required for objective setting else one can be lost their concentration and get derailed. When you have defined your objectives, you would not just feel certain about the work you are doing, however, you would likewise organize what needs are to be satisfied first. These raise your inspiration and confidence and you have an uplifting viewpoint towards the work that you are doing.

While defining objectives or notwithstanding making arrangements for them, you need to ensure that your objectives are

Savvy. That implies they ought to be:

Particular – i.e. to the point

Quantifiable – i.e. you can pass judgment on the amount of the objective is expert

Achievable – i.e. they ought to be inside your capability of accomplishment

Practical – i.e. they ought to be essentially achievable and not something which is obscure

Auspicious – i.e. there ought to be a time span in which these objectives ought to be accomplished

In this way, having a SMART approach while defining objectives would influence you to distinguish the escape clauses, check yourself and help you accomplish your objectives effectively. These objectives would enable you to climb the stepping stool of achievement in moderate yet solid advances.

inside a due date, set littler objectives which would enable you to accomplish your bigger objectives. For this situation, steps, for example, speculation, information accumulation, result examination, and gathering can be the littler advances which would accomplish the objective of report accommodation. Due dates ought to dependably be related with littler objectives as well so that as you cross them, you know about your advancement and the work is finished.

The real piece of objective setting is that it ought not to be unbending. Objectives ought to be set with the end goal that they are achievable and adaptable. Adaptability doesn't intend to be exceptionally tolerant of the objectives, but instead, you should liven up your objective arrangement as you oblige it. Stopping it up would make you remedy the issues which you look in the usage of your objective arrangement. In this way, time your objectives well, liven them up consistently and plan them as indicated by your needs with the goal that you don't wind up losing the diversion.

There are numerous kinds of objectives that you can set, for example, proficient objectives, imaginative objectives, individual objectives, family objectives, instructive objectives, budgetary objectives et cetera. By sorting your lifetime objectives, you would have the capacity to ensure that nothing is forgotten. Line up your objectives with the goal that you realize what to organize first and when to execute it.

Objective setting causes you to plan your life, as well as empowers you to guarantee that you are responsible for your life. Defining shrewd objectives along these lines guarantees their opportune finish and lessens your feelings of anxiety.

When you have an expansive objective to accomplish, ensure that you isolate it into littler objectives which appear to be anything but difficult to accomplish. For example, on the off chance that you need to present a critical report.

Chapter 3

The qualification among Objective and Values

You may discover intriguing to realize that everybody in this world is controlled by values. Our qualities and convictions are reflected through the choices we make to lead our lives successfully. We receive certain qualities from our family, here and there society or now and again we simply encapsulate them. Positive qualities can be embraced at any pace of life, ensure the incentive to seek after has a positive, solid and fundamental impact on your life. Since you move inside a general public it's important to uphold such qualities that meet the requests of society.

Preceding some other exchange, you have to know the contrast among qualities and objectives. Qualities are not objectives; in any case, they are between related with objectives and are exceedingly dependant on them. Objectives reflect targets while positive qualities frame the base of an effective life. You require some premise to lead your life, a few convictions, and deeds that drive and bolster the motivation behind your choices. Powerful qualities dependably impact your choices decidedly and enable you to pick the correct way to progress.

While managing our customers, we ensure he knows about the viability of positive qualities and is profoundly verbalized with them. Scribbling down the qualities is a decent method to safeguard them in our lives.

Thinking for approaches to kill your opportunity in brilliant radiant days, expounding on good and bad choices you have made in your past, considering the parts of fervor and inspiration in your life or contemplating about the activities that may add steadiness gives you edges to acknowledge what fact esteems have in your life. Additionally, you will be clear to separate among positive and negative qualities that impact your life.

You additionally need to realize that your scribbling of qualities ought to be in the current state rather in past, for example, express "I am steady fiscally" more eagerly than "I will be steady monetarily".

All you require is to arrange your qualities and scribble them as per your need. While composing I am steady monetarily, you can include different qualities like "I pay my liabilities on time, toward the month's end I am ready to spare some sum and I survey my protection frequently"

You can express your qualities to the zones of family, companions, network, ethics, instruction, vocation, wellbeing, accounts and diversion. Scribbling your qualities and further grouping them may require some serious energy however once you are through this course, you will without a doubt be clear about what your qualities are and how they impact your activities.

Try not to delay in offering time to recognize your qualities since they are the premise on which you set up your objectives. You turn out to be sure about what esteems have impacted your life decidedly and contrarily also. Now and again when you are in the condition of settling on a lifetime choice you certainly require a reasonable vision of your possibilities. You as of now have your qualities there in your psyche yet keeping in touch with them down on a bit of paper will without a doubt enable you to characterize them and set your needs in like manner.

Chapter 4

Why inspiration is critical for an effective life

Being fruitful is imperative for everyone. It is the inherent need of people to pick up acknowledgment, poise, and achievement. In any case, so as to succeed, one should be exceptionally energetic. This is so on the grounds that inspiration enables one the dormancy and to push themselves towards progress. Notwithstanding, inspiration is essential for progress because of different reasons too. A portion of these are a per the following:

1-   inspiration fills in as the fundamental startup:

Have you at any point been compelled to do some work that you don't care for? How have you responded to that function? Not that emphatically without a doubt! Presently contrast that work with some work that you jump at the chance to perform. do you understand the distinction in your disposition when you look at both of these errands? Which one was refined rapidly with a superior work quality? Obviously, the errand you preferred performing was performed way better. This is the thing that inspiration is. It fills in as a startup so you can excel with the work. The most troublesome part of an errand is to kick it off, and once things begin, there is no thinking back. In this manner, inspiration is a key factor in influencing you to begin on your approach to progress.

2-   inspiration makes you continue moving:

At the point when on the way of achievement, you are not generally compensated with progress. One needs to tumble down commonly before stretching up and moving beyond. Deterrents, all things considered, are a fundamental part to make you more grounded. It makes you deserving of your prosperity. In this way, you must be rationally arranged to confront the intense work, the difficulties and the issues in request to push forward. In this way, you have to keep yourself propelled so as to continue pushing and proceeding.

3-   Do something additional:

Would it be that the fruitful do that we don't? We have dependably pondered about this and found no solution. Its what they do 'additional' makes them fruitful. Regardless of whether you have begun up, moved one and confronted provokes, despite everything you have to push it past what your ordinary limit is. At exactly that point would you yield the product of achievement! Doing the important would take care of business at any rate, so what about doing that additional piece, with the goal that the errand itself would brag about who has done it! Consider it!

4-   It is exhausting without inspiration:

For what reason do you take books to peruse or tune in to music while going on a long voyage? It is to make you feel new all through the trip. Same is the situation with inspiration. The street to progress is long, exhausting and dreary, yet in the event that you have inspiration as your sidekick, at that point you require not stress over anything. Troublesome occasions can be helpfully continued by inspiration as being roused guarantees that you do not exclusively do it the correct way yet, in addition, live it up as you proceed.

So dependable feel spurred, keep your expectations high and look towards a more promising time to come.

Chapter 5

Personal development through inspiration

With a specific end goal to be glad and fulfilled, one should be roused. Inspiration fundamentally gives us the would like to look forward and dream higher. The power moves us to proceed. In any case, for what reason do we have to change? Individuals change for different reasons. Some change since they would prefer not to confront the agony in their lives. Some change since they are tired of their disappointments. For example, less than stellar scores can influence us to understand the significance of diligent work while considering and can propel us to change. Additionally, obligations can make us search for different employment or to accomplish in excess of one occupation.

This world is loaded with pessimism and paying little heed to whatever individuals say, we have to confront this antagonism and endeavor to get over it. In any case, it is you who needs to choose. Who is accountable for your life, you or your environment? When you conclude that you are responsible for whatever transpires, you will put your foot down and get over whatever cynicism encompasses you.

It is simple for us to remain is the asylum of our usual range of familiarity, yet have you ever had a go at venturing out of your customary range of familiarity and bring a sneak look into what lies past? What precisely keeps you from doing as such Disappointment ? Fears ? Disgrace ?

The fundamental thing that you have to enhance yourself is first, to have an objective and set a few targets. When you know where you are going towards, you will effectively keep up your concentration and not be strayed away by anything that prevents your way.

Next is to set some solid designs which can empower you to go for your objectives. While arranging, don't simply think inside your customary range of familiarity. Venture out of the crate so as to find a more up to date you. Recognize your issues and restrictions and utilize methods to get over them. Ensure that you realize what your shortcomings are and amend them while being in the area of the moral qualities that you treasure.

Execute your arrangement and don't stress whether you have succeeded or not. Disappointments would not break you, yet rather would fortify you. Revamp your plans on the off chance that they fall flat, recognize escape clauses and utilize techniques which enable you to defeat these provisos. Each disappointment shows you what to maintain a strategic distance from and closes in giving you a major exercise. Gain from these exercises with the goal that you can fortify the more up to date you.

Attempt to keep away from antagonistic musings and individuals. Such considerations and words keep an eye on self-restraint your potential and influence you to go feeble. On the off chance that you have confidence in your plans, you center around your bearing and roll out improvements just on the off chance that you wish to, paying little mind to what others say. This approach would make you hop over the impediments that square your direction.

In conclusion, you have to appreciate life and accept ridiculously. When you are glad and substance, your brain would work quicker and achievement will come to your direction. So hang on hard to your fantasies, take control of your life and set ahead to appreciate the voyage with a fresher you.

Chapter 6

Challenge your personality to be inspiration

The activity of having an objective situated conduct is otherwise called Inspiration. The real reason for inspiration is to diminish the psychological or physical pressure and to raise the factor of bliss in a man. Inspiration is for the most part of two kinds: Intrinsic and Extrinsic. The inherent inspiration is what is shown by the enjoyment or worry in the given action and is fairly inborn i.e. inside the individual itself. Despite what might be expected, outward inspiration is what is shown or improved by outer factors, for example, cash, prizes, endowments or terrorizing.

In the event that a man is unequivocally spurred to accomplish or gain something tremendous, at that point that individual is being associated with pointing high for what's to come. This is the inspiration behind why inspiration is interlinked with challenges. Also, our body – physically and rationally is composed so that it is constantly prepared to acknowledge and confront distinctive difficulties.

Inspiration can be clarified advance by one of the situations given underneath:

- If, for example, one comes to realize that they are in threat, at that point their prompt reaction takes all the vital measures keeping in mind the end goal to keep themselves from the peril and guarantee wellbeing.

The situation said above difficulties one's security and way of life. That is the reason it figures out how to rises ones inspiration towards the demonstration of securing themselves. In this way, we have to draw in ourselves in different difficulties with the goal that our spirit and inspiration remain supported. Confronting and conquering challenges has a tendency to grant a positive inclination that expands one's inspiration. It likewise makes you test your understanding and to what degree, you can extend yourself.

The most ideal approach to manage and include challenges in your way of life is to accept the day by day standard as a test and utilize it to change your character and considering. You can set day by day objectives and endeavor to achieve them effectively. A man's general character and identity are framed by means of learning and rehearsing the standards and estimations of the societal culture. In any case, every one of the qualities doesn't impact us. That is the reason one must have a right temper and inspiration with the goal that they can make their own particular qualities and live by them. In this manner, constant re-molding of your internal identity would give you a chance to see everything as a test and experience the difference in values that are required. An excess of unwinding of the mind would make you feel like a slowpoke so it is smarter to keep the cerebrum in real life.

It may tire keep yourself up to the difficulties constantly yet when you wind up accustomed to it, you would ace the aptitude of being inspired and effective.

Chapter 7

20 characteristics for an effective life

We regularly think about how a man can be so effective throughout everyday life! Is it since he acquired the achievement or is it in light of his one of a kind character? There are sure attributes that we can receive

with a specific end goal to be effective throughout everyday life. These are:

Truthfulness: Being genuine and following your qualities and convictions would promise you an achievement. So don't endeavor to be something that you aren't. Simply act naturally and inspire others.

Be authentic: Your activities are more prominent than your words. So don't misrepresent or cheat others. Simply be veritable.

Being wholehearted: You ought to be energetic with respect to things you do. So you ought to wholeheartedly give yourself to do great to other people and your locale.

Genuine: Being straightforward is very troublesome yet when you let trustworthiness manage you, you'll make more prominent progress. So never delude or do misrepresentation to excel throughout everyday life.

Sincere: Be straightforward and acknowledge others. Thank individuals who do great to you and contact those in require.

Generosity: Be warm and bona fide with others. This would emanate your character and fondness towards others.

Modesty: No issue how rich or effective you are, dependably be modest with others. This would longer affect others.

Individual uprightness: It is essential that regardless of how effective you move toward becoming, you ought to dependably keep your qualities flawless. Never exchange your ethical qualities for material advantages.

Ethical soundness: Be agreed and hold your ground to stick towards your convictions. Try not to give others a chance to degenerate you.

Practical insight: Show great and reasonable judgment throughout everyday life. Treat everyone with fairness and regard.

Concentrated: Always keep up your concentration and give your aggregate regard for the general population you collaborate.

Graciousness: Be great to other people and show affability even to the individuals who are outsiders.

Urban sense: Exhibit politeness and regard. Try not to rule individuals and talk with benevolence and regard.

Intelligence: Wisdom is picked up by involvement. Be in contact with your internal identity keeping in mind the end goal to increase higher comprehension and knowledge.

Philanthropy: Be liberal and magnanimous to other people. Stretch out help even to the individuals who have not helped you.

Sympathy: Know that everyone is unique and has distinctive requirements. Comprehend others sentiments and considerations.

Sensitivity: Always be thoughtful to individuals under passionate pressure. Endeavor to comprehend things from their perspective.

Humane: Reach out and help the individuals who are in trouble. You wouldn't trust the great wishes they'll convey to you.

Benevolence: Think for others without being narrow-minded. Do great and don't expect things consequently. Besides, don't express to others the favors you improve the situation them.

Decent: Give your cash, time and information to other people with the goal that they can gain from your experience. Try not to hold back reasoning that they'll stretch out beyond you. It takes a high personality and a liberal heart to do that!

The characteristics given above are a portion of the characteristics that a fruitful individual ought to have.

Attempt to embrace them in everyday life and make them a piece of your character.

Chapter 8

Stress administration

Stress is the additional pressure that we take which makes us experience various medical issues – both physiological and mental. Along these lines, it is critical to ease stress however much as could reasonably be expected. Stress administration is, in this way, the alleviation of stress that is imperative for everybody to know. A lot of variables can cause stress and in stress administration, the disposal of these activating components is as critical as different elements. A ton of research is being done in the areas of stress so more investigation with respect to stress administration should be possible.

Stress hugely affects the physical wellbeing. It can cause heart issues, pressure cerebral pains, weight reduction or even weight gain. There is no dependable result of stress on a man as various individuals respond contrastingly to it. Now and again, it can turn out to be very deadly as it can even reason cardiovascular assaults or strokes.

People are animals of extraordinary fluctuation. In this manner, their responses to stress administration additionally differ as it were. Every one of the strategies for stress administration probably won't be similarly compelling for every person. That is the reason one needs to find their very own instrument for reducing stress. Right off the bat, the reason for hidden stress ought to be assessed. Stress can be identified with work weight, family weight or any basic medical issue over which one has little control. Mates, kids or work companions can be the person who triggers the stress one countenances. Work issues, for example, stringent due dates, expanded outstanding task at hand, irritating manager, gibbering coworkers or a low pay would all be able to upgrade your stress levels. Along these lines, one needs to find their stress causing factor or various factors in order to have the capacity to control stress. It is adequate that multiple occasions, circumstances are not under your control but rather simply comprehending what factors makes you get stressed, can have a tremendous effect on what methodology you lighten it.

It is said that giggling is the best treatment for any ailment. In any case, one can't snicker constantly while in stress. That is the reason compelling strategies for stress administration ought to be contrived. A few people get pets which enable them to lighten stress. Some introduce drinking fountains or aquariums in their home keeping in mind the end goal to make the earth stress free. Some even utilize shout treatment, crushing delicate things, going for running or running, or taking up some interest with the goal that they can viably diminish and deal with the stress. Incredible physical exercises additionally tend to diminish adrenaline which can diminish stress levels found in a man. The last administration strategy to lighten stress is the utilization of prescriptions which are endorsed by an expert specialist. It is any way prescribed that all the stress administration procedures ought to be attempted upon before going for meds as these have a tendency to have heaps of symptoms on the body.

Along these lines, it is very essential that stress causing variables ought to be previously recognized and after that, mitigated by means of specific procedures. This would enable a man to battle this danger as well as one can keep them fit and sound for a more extended era.

Chapter 9

Time administration

In this quick-paced world, a typical protest that nearly everyone has is that they need time to get things done. Before, time administration was thought to be a thing related for businesspeople as it were. Be that as it may, these days, everyone falls under the space of time administration. Individual lives, and additionally work lives, are efficient once a man takes after the spaces of time administration. Time administration benefits ones mental and physical wellbeing and gives them a sheer feeling of control and fulfillment. Individuals who are responsible for their chance really tend to lead many satisfied and effective lives.

The procedures of time administration are not settled or inflexible. Additionally, it isn't essential that every one of the general population become acclimated to all the time administration strategies. That is the reason one needs to search for the system that best suits them with the goal that the affectivity is greatest. We as a whole tend to hone time administration somehow or the other. What should be centered around is the manner by which to amplify the adequacy of our strategies.

A few hints for time administration are given as takes after:

Set your objectives and destinations. This implies at whatever point you set out to accomplish something, you should comprehend what reason you need to satisfy. This would give you an ability to read a compass as well as help you allocate particular timings to whatever errands you need to achieve.

Set clear needs in your brain. You should realize what is more critical to you and what should be done earnestly. Organizing would enable you to survey your necessities and prerequisites in the long haul. A definitive accomplishment of a man relies upon how well he/she organizes things throughout everyday life. Here and now, and additionally long-haul needs, ought to be made which ought to be identified with each other. This will, in the long run, make you effective.

While organizing, be stern with those parts of your opportunity which are not adding to the long haul objectives that you have set for yourself. Expel these pointless territories from your opportunity zone with the goal that you can center your energies towards accomplishing more.

While mapping your convenient needs, make a point to incorporate family time and unwinding time in your everyday practice. This would guarantee great wellbeing and significant serenity. Additionally, a considerable measure of time for appropriate dinners and exercise in order to keep up a sound ordinary life.

Record your needs for a specific era with the goal that you can look at your weaker regions and fortify the time spent on them.

Continuously keep a journal to design each day, week and month, a lot of online organizers, programming, and so forth are currently accessible so you can get to your standard designs from home or from work without conveying everything that heap. Utilizing the regular dairy is better as it gives you a chance to get off the PC for a bit and think about your needs with a quiet personality. You can begin with gradual steps and influence a To schedule day by day when you begin your day. This can gradually improve your propensity for arranging you are everyday schedule while you design up slowly for the entire daytime organizer mode.

Time administration is without a doubt an additionally fulfilling approach to lead your life. This additionally causes you to be responsible for what you do and diminishes stress while enhancing well-being.

Chapter 10

Approaches to maximize your possibility

We are altogether invested with an extraordinary thing – i.e. our possibility. A few of us understand this possibility very from the get-go throughout everyday life while, for a few, it takes a lifetime to understand this. These last individuals who set aside an opportunity to understand their possibility frequently acknowledge the way that they have lost the time expected to convey their genuine possibility to surface. That is the reason, it is extremely essential to understand your possibility inside a given day and age, else its regularly past the point where it is possible to start. In addition, one can likewise understand their shrouded ability while finding their genuine possibility. This is finished with understanding, with the assistance of family, companions and even adversaries. In any case, tragically, individuals on occasion, likewise keep an eye on de-inspire a man to such a degree, to the point that their look for their concealed possibility winds up lost in their wretchedness. That is the reason we prescribe some broad rules which can be embraced keeping in mind the end goal to buff and clean your shrouded possibility.

1- Read books: If you need to find your concealed ability or possibility, you can investigate and look through your interests and remain side by side of the most recent happenings in your field of premium. This would keep you refreshed, as well as make you thrive particularly if your profession is to your greatest advantage fields.

2- Grow your introduction: You have to open your self to various happenings that occur nowadays. By and large, you will understand that your concealed possibility lies in the information that you were presented to since youth. So you should

travel to places, inquire about subjects of interests and make informal organizations with partners that may enable you to find your concealed possibility.

3- Find a decent coach: An effective guide who comprehends you would absolutely influence you to understand your shrouded possibility. They will help you with viewing matters, for example, managing family matters, business dealings, and different perspectives. A coach would absolutely achieve that concealed ability that you have not understood yet.

4-   Take testing work: Taking up difficulties would enable you to improve your possibility and discover it. Being out of your usual range of familiarity would not just influence you to acknowledge what you are made of, however, you would likewise be amazed to find those perspectives about your identity that are really obscure to you.

5-   Participate in rivalries: Participating in rivalries would enable you to take advantage of your own ability pool and find the unfamiliar! This would require you to expand your chance and vitality and improve your abilities.

6-   Try new things: you should regard each day as another day, a fresh start. Look forward at new roads and don't dither to attempt new things or going for broke.

Each one of us has remarkable possibility covered up inside them. We should simply to wake up and begin searching for them.

Chapter 11

Defeat Snags Created By Yourself - Restricting Beliefs

Snags don't need to stop you. On the off chance that you keep running into a divider, don't pivot and surrender. Make sense of how to climb it, experience it, or work around it. - Michael Jordan

Life is unquestionably troublesome that it is by all accounts. We tend to confront issues and snags in each period of our life. However, we know, that we need to look forward and pace up. The snags can be as family clashes, money-related issues, wellbeing related issues or issues identified with the change in social life. These are really identified with oneself constraining convictions that prevent us from pushing forward.

The premise of this issue is that the littlest observation can make a conviction which continuously becomes bigger. A lot of times, we have a tendency to wind up oblivious and have a tendency to coordinate every one of the activities as per these self-shaped convictions. These intuitive demonstrations have a tendency to gradually turn into a piece of our character and result in an enormous effect on our identity. When we discuss such convictions, these can be of different kinds. There are numerous convictions which have a tendency to positively affect our identity and way of life. Be that as it may, at times, these convictions can be adverse, which when fortified on our identity, have a tendency to make an immense effect and makes us frail.

When confronting such snags throughout everyday life, one needs to dependably manage persistence and mettle. The more grounded we confront these snags, the lesser they'll move toward becoming. There are likewise different approaches to manage these snags, for example, the accompanying:

1- Positive reasoning: This is the initial move towards addressing your issues. The plain idea of stopping an undertaking could never under any circumstance let you prevail by any means. That is the reason a positive attitude is required at all the occasions so as to discover an answer for the issues and snags you confront. Positive reasoning gives you a chance to have an unmistakable reasoning as well as makes you center around what you need to accomplish.
2- Relax your psyche: Tension and stress could never give you a chance to prevail throughout everyday life. Being sans strain would make you concentrate so most extreme hindrance is wiped out.

3-   Perseverance and industriousness: The issue would not comprehend without anyone else. Be that as it may, you have to sit tight for the outcomes to surface. This tolerance and continuance is an involvement in itself, which, through the trial of time, would influence you to have a radical new knowledge about the thought of the issue.

4-   Find new chances: Dynamism is the way to progress. So don't sit tight for chances to appear. Or maybe, assume responsibility and find new difficulties and openings in your day by day schedule work. It would make you imaginative, as well as would give you heaps of assurance and quality.

5-   Inspiration: The component of motivation is the desire or dream that makes you work harder and beat snags. Motivation gives the start that one have to impel ahead towards a higher future.

Chapter 12

Save work-life balance

The world is changing so quickly that each other individual currently needs to works keeping in mind the end goal to carry on with a superior life. In this race, one regularly tends to stir up their own and expert life. This outcome in a disordered up life, fouled up needs, an absence of time and generally speaking disappointment. This additionally gives an inclination to the individual that in spite of all the diligent work, one has as yet something missing throughout everyday life. This missing component is the psychological peace and serenity that one needs to focus on life.

It is along these lines fitting that one takes after specific guidelines so as to keep their lives simples, and carries on with a more advantageous existence with a harmony between the individual and expert life. A portion of these components is in your control while some might be out of the areas of your control. For accommodation, we'll take a gander at a few hints which are isolated into three perspectives beneath:

At work:

1-   Take little breaks amid the day. A ten-minute break can be taken at regular intervals so your adequacy and work profitability can upgrade.
2-   Prioritize your day and separation your opportunity reasonably.
3-   Limit all the email correspondence to the office as it were. Try not to take your pending work home.
4-   The refinement between the work and individual life ought to be kept independent. Try not to work or consider work all day, every day.
5-   Deal with implausible due dates previously it is past the point of no return. Impart the issues to your supervisor to keep away from issues finally.
6-   Consume your win leaves/travels with the goal that you can return new at work once more.

At home:

1-   Relax and invest energy with family in the wake of coming back from work.

2- Divide family unit tasks among relatives so that after all the work is finished, the family can sit together and share some quality time.

3- Exercise notwithstanding for no less than 10 minutes every day. It would invigorate you and you'll feel more stimulated.

4- Eat sound nourishment so you have the vitality to invest energy with your family and furthermore to work gainfully.

5- Adopt a diversion that you can seek after with your family or companions. This would keep your psyche off work and furthermore make you significantly more invigorated. Leisure activities are likewise very successful to lighten pressure so you can utilize a decent side interest and make utilization of it.

In people group:

1- Spend some quality time in your locale. Dedicate some willful time to network work with the goal that you can commit your cash, training and time to social work. This would upgrade your fulfillment level and furthermore present to you a feeling of social duty. You can likewise produce reserves, help in organizing corporate social obligations and utilize your greatest ability to serve your locale.

2- You can likewise partake in your youngsters' school occasions and parental social orders with a specific end goal to comprehend what your kid is realizing at school. Parental gatherings are likewise associated with sorting out capacities and social errands for the school kids. This would enable you to deal with your opportunity, as well as instill such social and extracurricular propensities in your kids.

Chapter 13

Managing Life Challenges

It is very notable for everything that everything begins with our psyche. The littlest idea is being produced into a thought, which takes the state of the activities keeping in mind the end goal to be executed. This entire procedure is being worked inside one's psyche with the goal that one can prepare. That is the reason inspiration is a critical reasoning methodology that all effective individuals have. We have all been liberally conceded with inspiration inside us, yet of course, it's a matter of decision for the individuals who need to utilize it or not. Individuals who are sure in their methodologies appear to draw in us more than the individuals who are negative and continually accusing things or their condition for the disasters.

Our manners of thinking are controlled by our mind which additionally reflects and is shown by our conduct, demeanor, and observation. It additionally demonstrates the kind of way of life we would lean toward. The individuals who are cheerful have a tendency to have positive reasoning which emanates around them. Notwithstanding, the individuals who are bleak have a negative atmosphere that transmits around them. Accordingly, it is dependent upon us concerning what sort of way of life we lean toward. Bliss and hopelessness, both are an essential component of life. Regardless of how rich one will be, one can positively never stay away from the bliss or the hopelessness. These issues which encompass us tend to make us more grounded inside as they show us about existence, about qualities and how to confront diverse difficulties that we go over in our day by day schedule. It is, for the most part, observed that those individuals who confront their life challenges decidedly have positive outcomes while those, who confront challenges with a negative disposition, normally wind up with the negative outcome. So what precisely should your approach be while confronting life challenges?

The following are a few hints which will manage you to enhance your day by day schedule and expand upon your internal identity:

- When confronting negative contemplations, attempt to transform them into positive ones. Keep in mind forget that you can control your contemplations, your musings shouldn't control the manner in which you live! So as opposed to grumbling and accusing others assess your choices. Think about the most ideal arrangement under the given conditions and follow up on them

- Don't hang out with antagonistic individuals. Or maybe, remain in the organization of the individuals who think decidedly. Talk or get directing with individuals who tend to think emphatically and are a wellspring of motivation for you.

- Find satisfaction in the straightforward things throughout everyday life. Make sure to view the less lucky and be grateful for what you have.
- Love yourself as opposed to faulting. Be thoughtful and regard others. Do little signals of graciousness, for example, a basic grin and hi to the guardian, helping the elderly, and so on. The positive signs you convey are met with energy accordingly which builds your fulfillment level.
- Help the sad individuals. Give some willful administration at a vagrant sanctuary or a nursing home. Invest energy with the hopeless and emanate your inspiration onto them.

Keep in mind forget, you get what you give. So dependably send signs of positive and offer would like to other people. Do recollect that when you give others motivation to grin for and would like to esteem, you'll likewise recover that ten times.

Chapter 14

Sides of human conduct to succeed

Inspiration is the reason which ingrains individuals to set out upon certain conduct that is enticing in nature. This powerful nature has a tendency to inspire individuals towards that specific errand, objective or target. Along these lines, inspiration is the power that drives an individual and moves them towards their goals.

To be inspired, one needs to adjust to certain standards of conduct that really convey the psyche to work progressively. In this manner, it is a perspective which isn't identified with one's identity, however, is somewhat received by a man, who is inherently spurred. There are sure parts of practices that have a tendency to impel a man towards being roused. These are Arousal of conduct, Direction of conduct and Persistence of conduct.

1-   Arousal of conduct:

This is the activating element that brings a difference at the top of the priority list. At the point when a man is inspired, he/she tends to begin contemplating the activities identified with what propelled them. These activities excite one's conduct in which certain activity designs are made in the brain of the individual who is persuaded. In this way, excitement is likewise the enactment of conduct.

2-   The course of conduct:

The course of conduct is the arrangement of one's musings and activity designs with the goal that an ability to know east from west is shaped. At the point when a man's practices are coordinated, he/she has a tendency to keep up their concentration towards their objective target. In addition, the course additionally keeps up one's musings towards that specific action plan.

3-   Persistence of conduct:

The determination is a vital component in inspiration as it guarantees congruity and solidness with respect to the activity designs. It additionally keeps up one's inspiration and furthermore proceeds with the objective accomplishment of the individual.

Other than these social perspectives, inspiration is additionally provided food by a few thought processes that are critical. These can be mental or physiological in nature which falls under Homeostatic thought processes, (for example, those essential for living. Eg: thirst, hunger, and so forth), Non-homeostatic intentions, (for example, protect looking for propensities, interest, and so on) and Social/Learned thought processes, (for example, endorsement, gratefulness, and so on). Homeostatic components are intrinsic and require not be supported accordingly. They are available as an inborn piece of one's tendency. Non-homeostatic components have a tendency to be influenced by the environment and can emerge because of the general perception. Be that as it may, social or educated thought processes are distinctive in each person as individuals have a tendency to act in an unexpected way, confront an assortment of circumstances and are molded ceaselessly by the general population and the circumstance they confront.

That is the reason each individual's reaction to these intentions is very unique, contingent upon their childhood, experience, and learning design. In this way, every individual reacts diversely when roused, which is displayed by means of the social viewpoints and the individual intentions. The key point to note here is that regardless of how you are adapted, dependably react decidedly in order to boost your potential and harbor your inspiration.

When you figure out how to control these conduct perspectives, you can assume the responsibility of yourself and alter sails as indicated by the course of your life moves you in. This would make you move effortlessly into the domains of accomplishment.

Chapter 15

The education Part in a fruitful life

Training is one of the essential standards on which one's prosperity depends. To comprehend the part of training and its effect on progress, one needs to initially see how they measure a fruitful life. A fruitful life can be designated by a man's riches, notoriety, vocation position, property, resources and the vast majority of all, their identity. While many contend that one need fortunes for progress and the individuals who are conceived with riches and resources are as of now fruitful, we do need to understand that being conceived with resources would not make us effective until the point that we end up being deserving of it.

So paying little respect to the reality whether you are conceived rich or poor, you have to center around how you can be fruitful and how you can keep up this situation of yours. Presently comes the inquiry, for what reason do individuals press on being taught with a specific end goal to be fruitful! Indeed, it is very basic. Training gives you the ability to read a compass, the learning, the aptitudes, and the center which is required with a specific end goal to be effective. Obviously, a great method of reasoning is additionally imperative the same number of, who has to prevail in their vocation ways have done as such in light of the fact that they used sound judgment. However, our choices, in the end, rely upon our instruction and are somehow influenced by our level of training and experience.

An informed business visionary and an uneducated business visionary have diverse methodologies, procedures and arranging inclinations. In addition, instruction makes you emerge among the others, gives you nobility and beauty. The odds of having better-paid occupations and shockingly better vocations are for the most part dependant on your level of instruction. School dropouts, for example, Bill Gates – Microsoft, Michael Cell – Dell PCs and Steve Jobs of Apple are a portion of the exemptions who were either so clever or persevering that absence of training didn't stop them to be fruitful. Be that as it may, following their way isn't everyone's lead of the diversion as we need to confront the truth instead of dream about special cases. In spite of not having a higher education, these men were so persevering and wise, that they are the present extremely rich people. Nonetheless, not every person can follow in the strides of these excellent men as we don't have the required knowledge or the fortunes so as to make it as large as them. Anyway, what precisely do we do with a specific end goal to make it as large? We can't simply take a seat and begin imagining.

The best activity in these conditions is to assume responsibility and get instructed. A Masters or any Professional degree is the way to progress as these degrees would find us in better-paying employment as well as make us deserving of it. Our identity and qualities would be formed by the training we get, which would assist us with dealing with the various business and corporate circumstances that generally abandon us confounded. In addition, our internal identity would likewise be reinforced by means of training as the qualities that our instruction would give us, would likewise assist us with portraying our self in a greatly improved manner to the general public.

So recall forgetting, the way to progress is great instruction as it changes our insight, values and our approach towards the best approach to progress.

Chapter 16

The social part in a fruitful life

Having an awesome companion circle and associating with individuals is an incredible method to push your life ahead. It's not generally that we go over individuals whom we get on well with. Be that as it may, having a functioning social life is a colossal method to keep you helped up. Investing energy with individuals makes your states of mind inspired, as well as improves your passionate prosperity, identity, and conduct. The key point to comprehend here is that one ought to make a ton of companions as well as rather, be companions with those individuals who are liberal and eager. Such constructive individuals have a tendency to have a considerable measure of positive impact in your life.

Notwithstanding, while at the same time making social associations, it is critical that we understand some social propensities that would be poisonous for our social relations and ought to be best maintained a strategic distance from. In such manner, a portion of the accompanying tips ought to be actualized while associating with the liberal group of friends:

1- Talk about inspiration and energy of others:

A decent social resource for all occasions is to discuss the social resources of others as much as you can. This would make you discover what rouses them and how they have a tendency to be so naturally propelled. You can talk about their interests and ask them for what reason they are so pulled in towards them. As you show signs of improvement at this ability, you will understand that now and again, you can considerably find someone's concealed possibilities that even they are uninformed of.

2- Don't cry:

Crying is a noteworthy push-away. It's an exceedingly negative sign, a red caution for those whom you associate with. In addition, it makes your group of friends disdain you. So make tracks in an opposite direction from this whimpering propensity. Despite the fact that you may imagine that you don't generally cry, individuals around you may be more touchy about this issue. Simply be more reluctant keeping in mind the end goal to acknowledge how much individuals around you experience the ill effects of your crying and how frequently you do it! Do comprehend that protestation and whimpering are two distinct things. You grumble when you smoothly expound on how something is unsuitable and how it should change. In any case, crying is an entirely unexpected situation.

3-   Don't brag:

Bragging may give us awesome bliss, support the self-image for a bit, however really has a tendency to be very adverse for our social life. Be that as it may, no one wants to be in the organization of a braggart and it frequently leaves a terrible impact on the general population you associate with. Just in the event that you are a humorist and are bragging of fun, at that point, it is certain to be taken in a carefree way.

Nonetheless, you likewise need a refinement among trustworthiness and gloating. On the off chance that you are genuinely informing others regarding your accomplishments, at that point, there is no requirement for you to shroud them. Or maybe, in the event that you really have a craving for enlightening others regarding something, at that point that gathered be bragging.

To assess yourself on these parameters and endeavor to pass judgment on yourself about where you turn out badly while associating with individuals. Adjust yourself and utilize these tips in order to appropriately collaborate with individuals and move towards a constructive individual change.

Chapter 17

Factors that make a person unsuccessful?

There have been numerous articles composed on the best way to be fruitful, however not very many of them refer to the factors that make you unsuccessful! With a specific end goal to be fruitful, there are sure factors that you unquestionably need to stay away from in order to guarantee achievement. A portion of these components are:

- False convictions: Any inaccurate thought that you have about something is a false conviction. The best component for progress is to relinquish false convictions by advancing over them and moving beyond. A little false conviction, for example, being unfortunate or not ready to discover work ought not to prevent you from searching for an occupation. To get over false convictions, one needs to escape their customary range of familiarity and acknowledge challenges with the goal that they can defeat their false convictions and proceed onward towards more up to date skylines.

- External control: A specific state of mind which is unequivocally connected with being unsuccessful is faulting everything to outside factors. For example, when one doesn't perform well in an exam, they accuse their educator or the earth around them. While effective individuals return to their interior locus of control where they trust that they are responsible for everything. They fortify themselves inside with the goal that they can confront whatever difficulties life tosses at them.

- Persistence and diligence: Successful individuals have a tendency to be diligent throughout everyday life. They tend to proceed with their diligent work until the point that they accomplish what they need. Losing trust rapidly are the indications of the unsuccessful individuals who don't stand up after they come up short. So be solid and tireless on the off chance that you wish to succeed.

- Inflexibility: Unsuccessful individuals are very unbending. They tend to adhere to their out of date ways and don't care for adjusting to evolving circumstances. In this powerful world, one should be exceptionally adaptable keeping in mind the end goal to be fruitful. You have to adjust to circumstances as needs be, take hardships and attempt distinctive techniques in the event that one falls flat.

- Improper arranging: Being gotten ready for your future would promise you the achievement. In the event that you have your own plans, you will keep up your concentration and head in the right measurement. The individuals who are unsuccessful don't design or regardless of whether they do, their plans are deficient. Along these lines, you should be arranged else you'll be cleared by everyone around you.

- Lack of fearlessness: Ever asked why the unsuccessful ones are in every case abandoned? It's all a direct result of the way that they do not have the certainty of exhibiting their thoughts before the supervisors. You ought to talk up, be imaginative and give thoughts with the goal that the general population around you understand that you are certain.

- Reminiscing about the absence of assets: A considerable measure of unsuccessful ones remain behind on the grounds that they imagine that they don't have the cash or the assets to get things done. Why remain behind? On the off chance that you are confirmed that you must be effective, you'll need to get things done without assets.

- Fears: These are not the feelings of dread of the dim or the stature, but instead these are the apprehensions which block your capacities to jump ahead towards progress. Albeit inverse, the dread of progress or disappointment can both thwart your way towards being effective so conquered your feelings of trepidation and begin pushing forward!.

Chapter 18

Criteria for idealizing fruitful individuals

In this world, we, as people, have heaps of desires and dreams. All through the phase of growing up, we have a tendency to romanticize enter individuals throughout our lives, who can either be our most loved film stars, sportsmen, educators, relatives or even government officials. This steady optimism leaves an effect on us and on occasion, our identity mirrors certain attributes of our goals which we have retained from them in the proper way of time.

So is there really a specific rule for idealizing individuals throughout our life? Would it be a good idea for us to arbitrarily glorify just anyone who loves us? Indeed, the thing is, that not all people are deserving of optimism. It additionally relies on how, we, as a man, would need to see ourselves. A hoodlum would dependably glorify his mafia pioneer, not the neighborhood cleric! Along these lines, on the off chance that we seek to be commendable and fruitful people, at that point we have to romanticize individuals who have the accompanying essential characteristics:

- Uplifting state of mind: An inspirational disposition makes us effective, as well as makes us open to every one of the open doors that come in our direction. Fruitful individuals have inspiration transmitting from them and they never let go of any chance. It is these moment openings that have made them climb their prosperity stepping stools.
- Esteem time: Successful individuals likewise esteem their chance. They are very much organized and got ready for the day. That, as well as esteem the season of others and, satisfy their due dates appropriately. While heading off to a gathering, they are dependable on time and very much arranged.
- Responsibility: Despite being high-daring people, effective individuals have a tendency to be responsible for their activities, victories, and disappointments. They don't accuse their condition or the general population, just on the off chance that any arrangement comes up short.
- Proactive: Being very much arranged is the key attribute of fruitful individuals. They are proactive in their activities and their uplifting disposition underpins their proactive measures.
- Imaginative: Creativity is the way to progress. Innovativeness gives you a chance to see new changes and work towards them. Every one of the pioneers gathered be inventive as their innovativeness rolls out them execute certain

improvements that are required for an aggregate turnover of an association's pace.

- Very much imparted: Good relational abilities are a critical resource of the effective people. Being knowledgeable in the verbal as well as the nonverbal relational abilities reflects colossally upon the identity of a fruitful person. Contacting others by means of correspondence can pull in many individuals towards you who may likewise bring more current chances.
- Strength: Being fruitful isn't easy. It takes a considerable measure of persistence and versatility as triumphs don't come without disappointments. The quality expected to stand up in the wake of coming up short is the genuine test that effective individuals experience. This implies versatility, as a quality, ought to never be ignored while choosing fruitful goals. A man can't be effective on the off chance that they haven't experienced any balances.

Previously mentioned characteristics are among only a couple of qualities that effective individuals have. Notwithstanding, these characteristics are very commendable and one can search for these attributes while choosing their standards.

Chapter 19

Factors behind the significance of inspiration for effective life

We as a whole realize what inspiration is and how it influences us. In any case, frequently, regardless of all the learning and mindfulness, despite everything we get befuddled by the idea of inspiration. So would could it be that causes all the disarray? For what reason do we neglect to absolutely comprehend inspiration?

All things considered, the fundamental capacity of inspiration is very basic. It is to give us satisfaction and to expel torment from our life. This is the essential thing on which all the inspiration al talks, sessions or books are based. What fluctuates is the sort of joy and agony that it has a tendency to give. This makes you read books and take sessions keeping in mind the end goal to acknowledge what strategies you should do so as to be persuaded.

So why precisely is 'inspiration ' the key factor behind our prosperity? Why not 'knowledge' or 'diligent work' for example? Without a doubt, inspiration must have something that it got this status. The genuine article is that at whatever point we need to play out an undertaking, achieve an objective or basically do some work, we require a specific moving element that would influence us to do that work. This 'impelling element' is inspiration. It is this inspiration that tends to influence us to satisfy the achievements and play out some work.

Presently the inquiry is: how does our mind feel propelled with a specific end goal to influence us to play out that undertaking? Essentially, there are three vital factors through which our mental capacities. These are:

1.   Conceptual.
2.   Perceptual.
3.   Emotional.

These three variables, when working together, impel us to do the errand. The calculated factor is dependable to shape certain convictions and reasons. Every one of the inspiration s we feel emerges in this district as once we shape a conviction about achieving something, we feel propelled towards that undertaking. The perceptual locale is included with the accumulation of tactile information. Once roused, we utilize this perceptual sense keeping in mind the end goal to identify with our inspiration and further increment it. The passionate district is included in our feelings, which might be fear, satisfaction, energy, dread or anything identified with the main job. Inspiration is additionally felt by the passionate area which at that point offers ascend to the components of fervor and satisfaction, which we feel when we are spurred.

This cycle of mind working reveals to us how our convictions and qualities control our inspiration. When we have set the correct methodology and outfitted with the correct convictions, we could never wander off from our propelled objective. A general run with respect to the arrangement of convictions is that one ought to dependably search for the positive things and discover positive convictions. Energy is an extraordinary supporter of inspiration and bliss and it duplicates the impact of inspiration. Hence, if our convictions are back up by the establishment of inspiration, at that point we would have the capacity to solidly maintain our inspiration.

To close with, inspiration is an advantage that is molded by our mind. It is in our control about how we condition our brain to be roused. In this manner, have sound and positive convictions which can create and make you feel spurred.